Leaky Gut Syndrome – Could This Be Why You Are Sick?

A Step-by-Step Path to Wellness

RON KNESS

Contents

Disclaimer

This publication is for informational purposes only and is not intended as medical advice. Medical advice should always be obtained from a qualified medical professional for any health conditions or symptoms associated with them.

Every possible effort has been made in preparing and researching this material. We make no warranties with respect to the accuracy, applicability of its contents or any omissions.

See your healthcare professional before starting any diet or exercise program!

Introduction

If you've been experiencing digestive issues recently, you could have a leaky gut. Leaky gut is just now starting to come onto the radar for doctors as more and more people are developing gastrointestinal and other disorders with no known cause. If you have frequent unexplained sickness, you could have leaky gut syndrome.

What it means is things are getting through the wall of the small intestine that aren't supposed to get through.

But let's back up for a minute and first explain the digestive process.

Your digestive tract begins in your mouth and ends at your anus. It's like a long, squiggly tube, sometimes wide, other times narrow. This tube is a mucous membrane, like your skin, but contained within your body instead of covering the outside of your body.

And like your skin, it acts as a protective barrier. In this case, it separates your body from whatever it is you have eaten or drank, and also from post-digestive material or fecal matter. Besides this, each section of this tube has its own special job to do.

Technically, what's *inside* the tube, is *outside* your body, even though we don't usually think about it that way. Because your digestive tract is somewhat like interior skin.

Starting to get the picture now?

One of the big jobs of your small intestine is to finish the digestive process by continuing to break down the food you have eaten into smaller and smaller particles. And then, it absorbs the nutrients from that food through your intestinal wall and into your bloodstream where the nutrients can be absorbed by cells and converted into energy.

And it has another big job, too. It's supposed to keep harmful stuff inside the tube, where it can't cause too much trouble for your immune system. Things like bad germs, toxins, and food particles that are still too big for your body to use.

To do this, your small intestine has to be permeable to some extent. It needs to be able to allow the nutrients you need, including water, to get into your blood stream so they can be used for energy production, cell repair, and other needed functions. You could say it's programmed to open the gates when the correct password is given. And only the good guys - the nutrients - have the password.

But sometimes, the lining of the small intestine gets damaged. Its communication pathways can fail and the passwords get garbled. The gates can get jammed open, or even jammed shut.

And that can turn into even bigger problems.

In this guide, you will learn about what the leaky gut syndrome is, its potential causes, and proposed treatments that might be able to not only relieve your symptoms, but make leaky gut a thing of the past. Let's get started!

What Is a Leaky Gut?

Leaky gut, or leaky gut syndrome, is not actually an agreed-upon medical condition. The medical term for it is intestinal permeability. When something is impermeable, it does not allow liquid to pass through, such as water. If something is permeable, it allows liquid to pass through, or leak through.

Complementary and alternative medicine (CAM) practitioners have developed the theory that a leaky gut, that is one which is overly permeable, releases various toxins, microbes, and even undigested food particles and other potentially harmful substances into the body, leading to illness. They have speculated that a leaky gut might be connected with a range of health issues, including:

- Acne

- Anxiety

- Arthritis

- Autism

- Autoimmune disorders

- Bloating

- Cancer

- Cardiovascular disorders

- Celiac disease

- Constipation

- Crohn's disease

- Decreased immune function

- Depression

- Diabetes

- Diarrhea

- Eczema

- Gas

- Heartburn

- Hypothyroidism

- Intestinal pain

- Inflammatory bowel disease (IBD)

- Irritable bowel syndrome (IBS)

- Joint pain

- Metabolic syndrome

- Mood swings

- Muscle pain

- Osteoporosis

- Psoriasis

- Psoriatic arthritis

- and more.

If we look at this list, some of these are symptoms of a leaky gut could also be connected to other gastrointestinal issues such as:

- Bloating

- Celiac disease

- Constipation

- Crohn's disease

- Gas

- Heartburn

- Intestinal pain

- Inflammatory bowel disease (IBD) and

- Irritable bowel syndrome (IBS)

So it is easy to see why it is often difficult to get to the root of the issue. We can also understand that what we eat and how it is digested is important in relation to diabetes and metabolic syndrome. For those of you who are not familiar with metabolic syndrome, it is five related conditions that are thought to be a precursor of insulin resistance, which is thought to be a sign of diabetes.

The five conditions that could indicate you have metabolic syndrome are:

- High blood pressure

- High cholesterol

- High triglycerides (a certain type of cholesterol)

- High blood sugar

- Waist roundness, that is, a 'spare tire' around your middle, which can often be a sign of being overweight, another common symptom amongst those with metabolic syndrome.

A diagnosis of metabolic syndrome is usually made on the basis of three of these factors being present. As the name suggests, something is going on with the metabolism. This starts to cause poor health, and could potentially be the way the body is using, or losing, the nutrients it is taking in, which could be the result of a leaky gut.

But is it really possible for our digestive tract to be connected to autism? New research has shown that autism might be connected to autoimmune issues and chemical imbalances that result, as well as the genetic components of autism that have already been researched.

Even though there is no specific diagnosis of leaky gut, doctors do know that certain things can affect the permeability of the intestines and throw the microbiome, that is, gut flora, out of balance.

These include:

- Overuse of antibiotics, such as nonsteroidal anti-inflammatory drugs (NSAIDs) like aspirin and ibuprofen

- Taking Proton-pump inhibitors (PPIs), which reduce gastric acid production

- A poor diet that damages the microbiome

- A poor diet that lacks the nutrients needed to maintain a healthy microbiome

- Too much sugar

- Genetically modified foods (GMOs)

- Stress

- Tap water

- Mercury, such as in canned fish

- BPA, such as in plastic bottles we drink from

- Pesticides

- Yeast infections (Candida)

Food-borne illnesses can also trigger leaky gut, including:

Norovirus, a highly contagious stomach bug passed from person-to-person through bodily fluids, such as saliva, vomit, diarrhea, and poor handwashing practices.

It is known as the curse of cruise ships because of frequent outbreaks and the ease of transmission in confined spaces.

Salmonella, which comes from contaminated or undercooked foods, such as chicken and eggs, and from certain pets, including turtles, birds, and handling pet foods and then not washing your hands carefully afterwards.

Giardiasis, from the parasite Giardia, the most common stomach parasite in the US. It comes from water contaminated with fecal matter.

There are many more food-borne illness, such as E. coli, listeria, cyclospora, shigella that can have a significant impact on your gut. Some of these will resolve on their own. In other cases, they may require antibiotics. In still other cases, doctors will give a broad spectrum antibiotic to cover all contingencies. The trouble with this is that antibiotics of any kind will change the gut flora, killing helpful bacteria as well as harmful ones.

Doctors prescribing antibiotics "just in case," or because pressured to do so by patients who insist on getting a pill of some sort when they go to the doctor, has given rise to antibiotic-resistant 'super bugs' and in some cases, serious damage to the microbiome. One recent study has shown that one course of antibiotics can kills off so many bacteria that the flora still haven't recovered two years later.

One of the most serious forms of damage is Clostridium difficile (C. difficile, or C. diff) colitis, which is an overgrowth of C diff bacteria in your gut. This bacteria releases toxins that attack the lining of the intestines.

Though relatively rare compared to other intestinal bacteria, C. diff is one of the most important causes of infectious diarrhea in the US.

The most common symptoms are severe abdominal pain and watery diarrhea, sometimes mixed with blood and pus, up to 15 times a day. Such extreme loss of bodily fluids can lead to dehydration and death. Another potentially fatal symptom of C diff is if the bacteria forms an actual hole in the intestine.

At this point, C diff can really only be treated via fecal transplant. That is, the feces from a healthy person is inserted into the colon of a person with C diff in the hope of rebalancing the gut flora. However, getting enough healthy feces for transplantation has proven to be a problem, demonstrating just how many American digestive systems are in poor condition.

Studies are bringing us closer to an understanding of just how sophisticated our gut is. For example, did you know that 90% of our digestion takes place in our small intestine, NOT in our stomach? Therefore, a leaky gut can have serious health implications if left untreated.

Now that we know what leaky gut is, what illnesses it is connected to, and a number of the potential causes of leaky gut syndrome, let's look at how it is connected to autoimmune disorders.

Leaky Gut and Autoimmune Disorders

CAM practitioners are pretty sure that leaky gut syndrome exists. What they don't know is what affect that permeability has on one's overall health. Gastrointestinal disorders can produce a wide range of symptoms, many of which seem unrelated to the digestive system:

- We would all love to be able to go to the doctor, get a definitive diagnosis, and be given a pill and told exactly what to do to cure ourselves. In the case of leaky gut, it is just one sign of many potential underlying medical disorders. On the other hand, it might be a chicken-and-egg issue. Is the leaky gut a result of the disease? Or the disease the cause of the leaky gut?

- While some of this might sound like weird science, until more research is done, CAM practitioners and mainstream doctors interested in the theory, and in nutrition and/or autoimmune disorders, have to work with patients to track their symptoms and note their diet, lifestyle and habits. In this way they can try to narrow down what might be causing the leaky gut and any other illness they might be suffering as a result from it.

- It is important to note that many of the illnesses on the list in the previous chapter that might be associated with leaky gut have an autoimmune component. That is, they involve inflammation, something irritating the body in some way, which will often cause the immune system to attack the body it is supposed to be protecting.

The theory is that the substances leaking from the gut are perceived as threats by the immune system, which goes into full defense mode due to the leakage.

According to the American Autoimmune Related Diseases Association, approximately 50 million Americans have some form of autoimmune disorder. More than 80 different conditions come under this umbrella. They include:

- Graves' disease (fast thyroid)

- Hashimoto's disease (slow thyroid)

- Rheumatoid arthritis (RA)

- Systemic lupus erythematosus (SLE, or lupus)

- Multiple sclerosis (MS)

- and many more.

It is important to note that 90% of RA and SLE cases are in women. In terms of MS, women are 3 times more likely to contract it than men. Is there a hormonal component? Or are women's diets literally diets, unnatural ways of eating that rely on artificial sweeteners and other chemicals in an effort to control or lose weight, which are really damaging their gut and metabolism?

Some of these autoimmune disorders have symptoms in common. While these diseases are generally viewed as separate conditions, they share common causes. One of the main ones is the immune system having a hard time distinguishing friend from foe, resulting in the body starting to attack itself.

As the body's primary defense against disease and infection, the immune system is connected to all other biological systems. As a result, the immune system being turned 'on' and staying on can cause damage throughout the body, resulting in what is termed chronic systemic inflammation (CSI). CSI confuses and damages the immune system even more, leading to even greater dysfunction.

Therefore, rather than try to treat specific conditions one at a time, a holistic approach that gets to the bottom of the inflammation and autoimmune response could clear up multiple conditions. For example, men with prostate disorders also tend to have coronary heart disease and arthritis. Is it possible that what is causing the hardening of the arteries (arteriosclerosis) is related to the arthritis and prostate issues? Since we know arteriosclerosis is triggered by inflammation, as is arthritis, it's perfectly possible it could be related to prostate problems as well.

Since we are what we eat, our diet is a key factor in our overall health. If we have a leaky gut, however, we are failing to get the nutrients we need and the food and substances we are taking into our body through the food and water we consume can literally be poisoning us and causing our own body to attack these "invaders", doing even more damage.

While the causes of autoimmune diseases are not fully known, many triggers have been identified, including:

- microorganisms, such as bacteria or viruses

- environmental factors such as pollution

- medications

- chemical irritants

- intestinal permeability

- food sensitivities

Unhealthy foreign bodies that look similar to healthy cells, can confuse the immune system and cause both to be attacked. Genetic predisposition - a family history of arthritis or heart disease, for example, seems to make a person more prone to developing these illness themselves.

As we learn more about genetic components of disease, it can be easy for people to become discouraged and think that they are doomed … that there is nothing they can do to avoid becoming ill. But the truth is making healthy choices can offset the genetic risks, making it less likely you will fall ill.

One of the best ways to prevent a disease is to know its causes, and take action to counteract them. Even if you can't prevent the disease, knowing the signs and symptoms can help you spot the condition early so it doesn't progress into something serious that will be much harder, if not impossible, to treat. Let's look in the next chapter at the signs and symptoms of a leaky gut.

Leaky Gut Signs and Symptoms

There are a number of signs and symptoms of a leaky gut. Many of them are linked to gastrointestinal issues, as to be expected, but some are more general overall health issues. They include:

- Digestive issues such as gas, bloating, diarrhea, constipation

- Irritable bowel syndrome (IBS)

- Depression

- Fatigue

- Fever

- General malaise (feeling ill)

- Seasonal allergies

- Asthma

- Muscle aches

- Inflammation such as redness, heat, pain, and swelling

- Hormonal imbalances such as pre-menstrual syndrome (PMS) or Polycystic Ovarian Syndrome (PCOS).

- Celiac disease

- Crohn's disease

- Diagnosed chronic fatigue syndrome (CFS)

- Diagnosed fibromyalgia

- Mood disorders such as depression and anxiety

- Attention Deficit-Hyperactivity Disorder (ADHD) or Attention Deficit Disorder (ADD)

- Skin issues such as acne, rosacea, eczema or psoriasis

- Diagnosis of candida overgrowth (yeast infection)

- Food allergies, sensitivities and intolerances, such as to gluten

- Diagnosis of an autoimmune disease such as:

- Rheumatoid arthritis

- Hashimoto's thyroiditis

- Lupus

- Psoriatic arthritis

It's important to not try to relieve one symptom at a time, but rather, look at the problem holistically. Let's take a quick look at what you need to know about your digestive tract so you can grasp the potential effects of a leaky gut.

What You Need to Know About Your Digestive Tract

You probably take your digestive tract for granted, but it is an amazingly complex system with varied functions that extends from your mouth all the way to your anus.

You start digesting the moment you put food into your mouth. Your teeth and saliva start breaking down the food so it can travel down the esophagus to the stomach. Think of your digestive system as a finely-tuned conveyor belt, with the muscles within your stomach and intestines moving the food along to each important stage of digestion. This movement is called motility.

In the stomach are acids that digest the food even further so your small intestine will be able to remove the nutrients from the food and send them out to the rest of the body. The large intestine, or colon, will help get rid of the rest as waste products, which are removed through the process of urination (elimination) and excretion (stool, feces, excrement).

Digestive juices contain enzymes that break food down into different nutrients. The small intestine is responsible for 90% of your digestion, so a leaky gut can be a disaster for the body. In addition to releasing toxic substances, it will fail to transfer nutrients. Without essential nutrients, you will become ill.

The walls of the small intestine allow the nutrients to pass into the bloodstream, which delivers them to the rest of the body. Therefore, we know the small intestine is permeable.

However, if it is too permeable, your gut can leak into the body cavity. Hormone and nerve regulators control the digestive process, for example, signaling when you feel full, and when to release insulin.

Your food traveling from your mouth to your anus is a long journey of nearly 70 yards that involves a range of enzymes and digestive juices and about 1,000 different bacteria, many of them helpful, some of them harmful if they get out of control, such as C diff.

On such a long and complicated journey, a lot can go wrong. Therefore, taking a closer look at what you put in your mouth is the best way to decrease the risk of leaky gut and increase your digestive health. Let's look in the next chapter at foods that doctors believe contribute to leaky gut syndrome.

.

Foods Linked to a Leaky Gut

There are a number of foods and other things we consume that can be linked to leaky gut.

- Cow's milk and products made from it

- Whole grain wheat

- Glutens

- Genetically Modified and Hybrid Foods

- Tap water with chlorine and/or fluoride

- Sugar, and items that are perceived as sugar by the body

- Artificial sweeteners

- Artificial colorings

- Salt

- Preservatives

- Too much yeast in the diet

- Alcoholic beverages

Due to the food industry in the US and developed nations, many of these items are in the foods we eat without us even realizing them. Labels can be confusing and the manufacturers know all the loopholes. Cow's milk is used for taste and moisture. It's also powdered and therefore highly concentrated, and is used in all sorts of foods as a thickener.

So too is wheat, and the protein from the wheat, gluten. If you've ever tried to eat low-carb, you will know how hard it can be because wheat and carbs, like sugar, are everywhere and are often disguised as something else. Gluten is often labeled as food starch or modified food starch.

GMO and other engineered foods are bred to be sturdier, yield more, and be insect-resistant. This undoubtedly affects their make-up and digestibility. So to do the pesticides that are used on them and the water that helps grow them.

Some nutritionists term processed cane sugar "white death" because of its damaging effects on the body. This has led people to turn to what they think are healthier alternatives, such as honey, agave nectar and brown rice syrup. They are mistaken. The body still treats them as sugar. And brown rice syrup is heavily contaminated with arsenic, due to the water in the rice paddies where the rice grows being contaminated.

Artificial sweeteners are all man-made using chemicals. Stevia is a natural sweetener that is said to be safe and is far sweeter than sugar. In its natural form, it looks, smells and tastes like alfalfa. Unfortunately, this means it's not that versatile, so it gets heavily processed to make it look like white sugar.

Artificial coloring is yet another source of chemicals in the diet. Just think of the colors of Jell-O, Fruit Loops cereal, or Kool-Aid and you will get an idea of just how full of chemicals convenience foods can be, and what America is feeding the younger generation, or even eating themselves.

Salt makes food taste better. It is also used as a cheap preservative, for example, in cold cuts, cheeses, and smoked products such as salmon, bacon and ham. Cold cuts also have other preservatives such as nitrates and nitrites. Aim for low sodium foods.

Alcoholic beverages are created via yeast turning sugar into alcohol. Both the sugar and yeast have been linked to leaky gut.

Now that you know several of the most harmful foods in relation to leaky gut, what can be done to improve your digestion? Let's look at probiotics in the next chapter.

Probiotics Verses Preboitics

In recent years, more and more people have started to understand the importance of probiotics for the digestion. Bacteria in the digestive tract help digest the food and keep the intestine healthy. These bacteria are commonly referred to as gut flora.

However, gut flora can be disrupted and even killed off due to certain food and medications, in particular, antibiotics. Antibiotics have been overprescribed in recent years, with increasingly serious consequences.

Probiotics can help restore the balance and prebiotics are what they live on. Increasing attention is now being paid to the best prebiotics to help the probiotics do their work.

Prebiotics

Prebiotics should be part of a balanced diet. However, a lot of people have adopted a low-carb diet, or a gluten-free one, thus eliminating one of the main sources of prebiotics, whole grain wheat. But there are other options that are not grain-based, including:

- Artichokes

- Asparagus

- Bananas

- Chickory

- Garlic

- Leeks

- Onion

- Potatoes

- Soy beans

Probiotics

Lactobacillus acidophilus and Bifidobacterium lactis are recommended for maintaining gut flora. They can be found in Greek-style yogurt, and in kefir, a fermented dairy drink. Just watch out for a lot of added sugar in these products.

Some people buy expensive probiotics in the refrigerator section of a good health food store, but there's really no need to when yogurt is so cheap.

Avoiding antibiotics is another aspect to the importance of the probiotics as an essential part of healthy gut flora.

So, what can you do to recover from leaky gut syndrome? Let's look at some all-natural ways in the next chapter.

Recovering from a Leaky Gut

There are a number of steps that can help you recover from a leaky gut. They are known as the 5 Rs; they are:

1. **Recognize** the symptoms

2. **Remove** foods and factors that damage the gut

3. **Replace** the damaging foods with healing foods

4. **Repair** your leaky gut with specific herbs and supplements

5. **Rebalance** your gut flora with prebiotics and probiotics and helpful enzymes

Recognize

Determine whether or not you have leaky gut. Unfortunately, at this point there is no test for it, and indeed, many doctors won't even look for it as an explanation. Trust your knowledge of your own body. If you've been feeling drained, lacking in energy and generally feeling unwell, clearly something is going on. In which case, it's time to recognize there is something wrong with your health, and it's time to track what's going on, and make a change.

Once you've recognized there is an issue, it's time to try to resolve it. The best place to start is to remove foods that might be causing issues. You might consider fasting for a day or 2 and then reintroduce them one at a time.

Working with an allergy specialist can help. So could a nutritionist and a CAM practitioner such as a DO.

Different diets can help with leaky gut as well as a number of eating lifestyles changes that might help cure leaky gut.

Clean eating

Clean eating is latest buzz phrase among health-conscious consumers and emphasizes eating healthy, whole, unprocessed foods. It's like getting back to basics, eliminating all convenience foods and cooking from scratch. They will cook their food in such a way as to get maximum nutrition from it, such as making soups and stews and steaming food lightly.

Raw diet

In a raw diet, as the name suggests, you don't cook your food in any way. Instead, you consume a lot of vegetables, fruits, seeds and nuts all in their natural state – raw and uncooked.

Organic diet

In some cases, people go organic, buying only products which are certified organic because they will not be exposed to pesticides, commercial fertilizer, and other chemicals that might get absorbed into the food and then into the body.

Buying organic can be expensive, but shopping in warehouse clubs and growing your own food can help keep costs down.

Gluten-free

Many people are going gluten-free. Gluten is a protein found in wheat, rye and barley. It is like the glue that holds the food together. The food industry uses gluten for texture and consistency or 'mouth feel' of food. You will often see it on labels as starch or modified food starch.

The Anti-inflammatory diet

Another promising way to deal with your leaky gut is to try an anti-inflammatory diet. This has been shown to be effective in relation to medical conditions that manifest with extreme inflammation, such as arthritis. If an anti-inflammatory diet can help arthritis pain, it could well be worth a try for your leaky gut.

There are two main principles to an anti-inflammatory diet. The first is to avoid foods believed to cause inflammation. The second is to add foods to your diet that are known to relieve inflammation. Swapping the good foods for the bad can keep you satisfied instead of miserable and deprived. They are tasty and could even help you lose weight.

Your food journal

Many people with health issues keep a journal of symptoms and actions, so they can see if what they are eating, for example, has any effect on the way they feel. A food journal is a great idea if you think you have a leaky gut. Eat as you normally would for your first couple of days. Then fast for a couple of days, such as doing a juice fast with carrot and other juices, or a soup fast with bone broth or other clear homemade soups. Then start your anti-inflammatory diet, making changes and note down your results for each.

Here are some foods to swap out and some to add to your anti-inflammatory diet:

Foods to Avoid

1. Sugar and sugary foods like honey, agave and brown rice syrup, and fructose, such as high fructose corn syrup

2. Salt, commonly listed as sodium on food labels

3. Standard cooking oils such as corn, safflower and vegetable oil

4. Red meat such as beef and lamb, game meats like bison, boar and venison, and organ meats, such as heart, brains, kidneys and liver (all connected with gout, a very painful form of arthritis)

5. Processed meats/cold cuts such as sliced roast beef or ham, because they are full of salt and chemical preservatives

6. Refined carbohydrates such as cake, cookies and candies, white bread, white pasta

7. Full-fat dairy products such as milk, butter, cream, cottage cheese, yogurt and soft cheeses. Note that cheese can be high in salt as well, which is used to preserve it.

8. Artificial sweeteners and flavorings, such as aspartame (NutraSweet, Equal), and Monosodium Glutamate (MSG)

9. Alcohol, due to the inflammatory effects on the body, plus chemicals, such as sulfites that are used to preserve and stabilize wine

10. Trans fats, that is trans fatty acids.

There are two types of trans fats found in foods: naturally-occurring and artificial trans fats. Naturally-occurring trans fats are produced in the gut of some animals and foods made from these animals, such as milk and meat products.

But the main source is man-made, that is created artificially through the process of adding hydrogen molecules to liquid vegetable oils in order to make them more solid.

Trans fats are commonly labeled as partially hydrogenated oils. They are added to convenience foods like cookies, crackers and other snacks to make them shelf-stable so they won't spoil. They also add texture and what is termed "mouthfeel" to these foods in order to make them tastier.

Foods to Add to Your Menus

1. Olive oil (Extra virgin if you don't mind the stronger taste) – while it is a good fat, it still should be used sparingly, but it has no cholesterol. Regular olive oil can be used as a substitute for most recipes calling for butter or margarine

2. Cherries, sweet, and tart (highly recommended if you have arthritis)

3. Walnuts and other tree nuts (if you are not allergic)

4. Bell peppers, such as green, red and yellow

5. Ginger, fresh root or dried - great in Indian and Chinese food

6. Turmeric, fresh root or dried- great in Indian food and rice dishes

7. Berries such as blueberries, raspberries and strawberries

8. Probiotics, such as yogurt with live cultures and kefir, a cultured and fermented beverage made from dairy

9. Salmon and other fatty fish with Omega-3 fatty acids

Salmon is just one fatty fish rspich in Omega-3 fatty acids, which are said to be heart-healthy and reduce inflammation.

Popular fish include:

- Alaskan Salmon, wild, not farmed-raised

- Arctic Char

- Atlantic Mackerel

- Bass

- Catfish

- Flounder

- Haddock

- Halibut

- Herring

- Pollock

- Red Snapper

- Sardines

- Sole

- Swordfish

- Trout

Some of these species can have more than 1,500mg of Omega-3 per 3-ounce serving. The daily allowance is 2,000mg for ordinary people, up to 4,000mg for athletes.

Here's a handy chart of Omega-3 content in mg per 3-ounce serving: http://www.seafoodhealthfacts.org/seafood-nutrition/healthcare-professionals/omega-3-content-frequently-consumed-seafood-products

Other sources like shark, king mackerel and tilefish are rich sources, but tend to be high in mercury and other toxins, so eat sparingly.

Fish can be expensive, so check your local warehouse store. Steer clear of anything with a lot of breading on it or salty sauces.

Not crazy about fish? Non-fishy sources of Omega-3 includes:

- canola oil

- flaxseed - a tiny, crunchy, nutty seed that adds taste and texture to salads and baked goods

- flaxseed oil

- mustard seeds and greens, with the seeds used in Indian cooking and the greens boiled up like collard greens

- pumpkin seeds

- soybeans (tofu, edamame)

- soybean oil

- spinach

- walnuts

- wheat germ (found in whole grain wheat)

You can also get Omega-3 fatty acid supplements. The recommended daily allowance is 2000mg, so try to get it mainly from the food you eat. There's no need for mega doses. In fact, too much has been linked with heart health issues.

Fish oil supplements can also be expensive and not always very pure. Look for US or Canadian products. Krill oil and salmon oil should be very pure, safe and with the highest levels of Omega-3.

Green leafy vegetables and cruciferous vegetables

All vegetables are good for us because of the fiber and moisture helping us feel full, but there are a couple of classes of them that are most beneficial, green leafy vegetables and cruciferous vegetables.

Green leafy vegetables

There's a craze for kale these days as a green leafy food. It's being put into everything from soup to snacks. But there are lots of other options, some with an even better nutritional profile than kale. Add these to your menu too:

- Beet Greens

- Chickory

- Endive

- Iceberg lettuce

- Napa Cabbage

- Parsley

- Radicchio

- Romaine Lettuce

- Swiss Chard

- Spinach

Cruciferous vegetables

Cruciferous vegetables take their name from the cross shape they tend to grow in. Here are some tasty ones you will find easy to add to your meals. They are also quite filling and full of flavor, so they may help you lose weight.

- Arugula - this has a spicy, peppery taste and is great in salads

- Bok choy (Chinese cabbage, great in stir fries)

- Broccoli

- Broccoli rabe

- Brussels sprouts

- Cabbage

- Cauliflower

- Collard greens

- Daikon (Japanese radish, nice with fish)

- Horseradish, such as in shrimp cocktail sauce

- Mustard seeds, such as black mustard seeds (often used in Indian cooking)

- Mustard leaves

- Radish

- Rutabaga (Swedish turnip, or swede, orange in color)

- Turnips, root and greens

- Watercress-this has a peppery taste and is great in salads and with egg salad sandwiches

Vitamins and Minerals

Since leaky gut affects the absorption of nutrients from your food, it can start to lead to deficiencies, which can in turn worsen your leaky gut, creating a vicious cycle. When planning your meals, try to focus on natural sources of the following nutrients.

- Vitamin A

- Vitamin B, including B12

- Vitamin C

- Vitamin E

- Magnesium

- Iron

- Zinc

Here are a few suggestions regarding the main sources for each:

Vitamin A

Vitamin A is fat soluble, so it can be stored in the body. If you are looking for natural sources, think deep green, or orange foods.

- Butternut squash

- Beef liver

- Cantaloupe

- Carrots

- Kale

- Mangoes

- Pumpkins

- Spinach

- Sweet potatoes

Vitamin B, including B12

B vitamins are important because they are water-soluble, which means they can't be stored in the body.

They are also important if you smoke cigarettes or are under a lot of stress, because these make you use up B vitamins even faster. B can also be tricky because they are an entire family of vitamins from B1 to 12. The most notable ones are

- Vitamin B1   (thiamine)

- Vitamin B3   (niacin)

- Vitamin B5   (pantothenic acid)

- Vitamin B6   (pyridoxine)

- Vitamin B7   (biotin)

- Vitamin B9   (folic acid)

- Vitamin B12 (cobalamins)

B9

The most well-known is probably folic acid, since it is connected with healthy pregnancies. Main sources of B9 are:

- Asparagus

- Avocado

- Beans, such as black-eyed beans

- Broccoli

- Lentils

- Lettuce

- Mango

- Oranges

- Spinach

B12

B12 is not well-absorbed when a person suffers from leaky gut.

Mains sources of B12 include:

- Fortified cereals (but watch out for too much sugar)

- Mackerel

- Milk

- Salmon

- Sardines

- Soy (tofu, edamame)

- Swiss cheese

- Yogurt

It is important to note that excessive amounts of B9 and B12 in pregnancy have recently been linked with a significantly greater risk of autism, so remember, supplement, but don't overdose or treat vitamins as if they are a substitute for a healthy diet.

Vitamin C

Vitamin C is also water-soluble, so you need to replenish your supply every day. Fortunately, this is pretty easy to do, with a range of tasty foods. Here are a few natural sources:

- Bell peppers, yellow

- Berries, such as strawberries

- Broccoli

- Guava

- Kale

- Kiwi fruits

- Oranges (try to focus on the fruit, not a lot of juice)

- Papaya

- Peas

- Tomatoes

Vitamin E

Vitamin E maintains the walls of your cells and keeps skin healthy. It might contribute to maintaining the gut so it doesn't leak.

- Almonds

- Avocado

- Broccoli

- Kale

- Nuts like peanuts

- Olives

- Parsley

- Papaya

- Pumpkin seeds

- Spinach

- Swiss chard

Magnesium

Magnesium is an essential mineral used in many bodily function. Top sources include:

- Avocados

- Bananas

- Brown rice

- Dark chocolate

- Low-fat dairy

- Dried figs

- Mackerel

- Pollock

- Pumpkin seeds

- Soy beans

- Spinach

Iron

Iron is essential for healthy blood and circulation. Top sources to try include:

- Beans

- Beef or chicken liver

- Broccoli

- Clams

- Halibut

- Haddock

- Lentil

- Oysters

- Pumpkin seeds

- Spinach

- Salmon

- Sardines

- Spinach

- Tofu

- Tuna

- Turkey

Zinc

Zinc is required by many tissues and bodily functions. It also works in conjunction with magnesium to keep the brain sharp, which can help those with leaky gut who complain about a brain fog. Main sources include:

- Almonds

- Baked beans

- Beef

- Cashews

- Cheese, Swiss

- Chicken

- Chickpeas

- Crabmeat

- Flounder

- Kidney beans

- Oatmeal

- Peas

- Pork

- Pumpkin seeds

- Yogurt

A good multivitamin can help cover anything missing from the food you eat, but again, don't overdo it, as too many vitamins and minerals can lead to overdose and other health issues. An age-related formula like Centrum Silver for seniors can also help keep you in balance. You can buy many types relatively inexpensively through a warehouse club.

Reducing stress

One other really key aspect to improving your digestive health is to reduce stress in your life. There are a number of ways to relieve this and thereby improve your health - body, mind and spirit. Here are 15 top ones to try:

- Set priorities. Focus on what's important and let go of the other stuff.

- Identify tasks you can share or delegate, then ask for help. Don't try to do everything yourself.

- Get organized. Disorder can eat up time and make things tough to remember.

- Don't try to multitask. There's no such thing. It is just your brain switching back and forth between tasks. This leads to a lot of stress. Things take twice as long to do in the end compared to just doing one thing at a time from start to finish.

- Set short-term goals you can reach. Then reward yourself when you meet them with something fun and relaxing.

- Learn how to say no gracefully but firmly so you don't overextend yourself. Only agree to obligations that align with your priorities and inner truth.

- Maintain a positive attitude. Choose to look for the good in others and yourself. Choose to make the best of any challenge you face rather than looking on the dark side.

- Avoid perfectionism. Remember, things don't have to be perfect. Sometimes "good enough" is just fine.

- Set aside some time, even 5 to 10 minutes, for yourself each day, to just sit and do nothing, or do something you love.

- Laugh more. Look for humor in your everyday life, or watch a funny movie.

- Listen to music. Choose tunes that relax or make you feel uplifted.

- Get things off your chest. Talk to a counselor or a friend.

- Get regular exercise. Find something you like doing that you can work into your schedule.

- Eat well. You can't put in your best performance if you're running on an empty fuel tank.

- Take a time-out for meditation, visualization, mindfulness, deep breathing, yoga, tai chi, and other stress-relief techniques.

Meditation

Meditation is a practice in which an individual trains their mind, or induces a different mode of consciousness, with the goal of either achieving a particular benefit, or clearing their mind from a lot of the 'clutter' that can prevent them from living their best life.

There are different forms of meditation. Some attempt to empty the mind of all conscious thought. Other forms encourage contemplation of a particular topic, such as the nature of human life. Still others encourage visualization.

Visualization/Guided Imagery

Visualization means to summon up a mental image, to see it in the 'mind's eye', as the common phrase goes. Research has shown numerous benefits to visualization, also referred to as guided imagery. Benefits include controlling pain, getting ready for athletic or other kinds of performances, relieving stress and anxiety, and more. Guided imagery can transform a negative mindset to a positive one, and therefore alter mood and perceptions.

Meditation and visualization are therefore two methods of training the mind to relieve stress and can be done separately or together.

Mindfulness

Mindfulness is a form of awareness in which you focus on the present moment. It can be used in meditation and visualization.

Most people live in the past, hung up on things that happened to them that they feel they can't move beyond. They also live in the future a lot of the time, making plans for their careers, families and so on, even though no person has any guarantee that they will even be alive tomorrow. As the saying goes, everyone dies with a to-do list.

Mindfulness enables you to slow down and live in the present for a short time. It also helps improve your focus so you can be present in each moment, such as when you are spending time with loved one. If you're washing the dishes, focus on the task as if it is the most important thing in the world. If you're spending time with loved ones, be mindful, and you will see that 30 minutes together can be more meaningful than hours in the same room not connecting with each other.

Deep Breathing

Deep breathing is one way to relax and slow down the body, or energize it. Short breaths when you are stressed make you ready for 'fight or flight'. Long, deep breaths help you become steadier and give you time to make a thoughtful decision rather than react on the spur of the moment.

It can be used on its own, or as a preliminary to meditation and/or visualization. Deep breathing is also part of yoga, which can be a great stress reliever.

Yoga

Yoga is a combination of meditation, visual imagery, deep breathing and physical movement and postures. It also teaches you to be mindful, such as of your body. All forms of exercise can relieve stress. Yoga uses your own body weight to tone and trim. It increases flexibility, lowers blood pressure, and promotes better sleep.

Tai chi

Tai chi is a martial art which is low impact and slow and meditative. It is great for improving the circulation, balance, strength and flexibility.

Quality Sleep

One final stress-relief technique is to aim for high-quality sleep. Every adult should have 8 to 9 hours of sleep per night. Quality sleep also means Rapid Eye Movement (REM) sleep, a deep form of sleep that helps you rest and rejuvenate more efficiently.

A balanced diet, stress relief, exercise and a good night's sleep are all foundations of a healthy lifestyle and disease prevention. They can also help strengthen the digestive system and maintain the permeability of the gut.

One other important aspect is to maintain proper nutrition and regulate your eating habits. Treat your food as fuel. Crash diets, anorexia and bulimia can all have serious consequences, just like overeating.

CAM practitioners who have been investigating leaky gut have several suggestions for herbs and supplements that might be able to help with a leaky gut. Let's look a few of them in the next chapter.

Herbs and Supplements

There are a number of herbs and supplements that have been suggested as able to help a leaky gut. Many of them focus on healing and firming up the gut in order to increase its impermeability. Suggestions include:

Aloe Vera

Aloe vera is a healing plant often used to treat cuts, scrapes and burns. It is a spiny plant that can be grown almost anywhere, even in your home. When the spikes are cut, they exude a clear thick liquid/gel which can be applied to the skin. There are a number of drinks available on the market, but watch out for sugar. You can grow it yourself and add the gel to water or fruit juice in order to enhance internal health and healing.

Butyrate

Butyrate comes from the Greek for butter, so it will give you an idea of the main source of this particular fatty acid that promotes healthy digestion in the small and especially the large intestine.

We all know fiber is supposed to be healthy for us, but it will work best in the right microbiome. You could consume more butter or goat cheese, but they will have an impact on your cholesterol levels. There are supplements, but they are expensive and poorly absorbed.

A better plan is to eat foods that encourage your body's own production of butyrate. These include:

- Dark leafy greens

- Vegetables

Insoluble fiber

Usually found in grains such as:

- Amaranth

- Buckwheat

- Millet

- Oats

- Quinoa

Low-fat dairy with active cultures can also help. Some experts also suggest coconut water and kefir. Fermented vegetables like kimchi (Korean pickled vegetables) and sauerkraut can also help.

These foods not only boost the microbiome, they decrease inflammation, offering double the benefit for the same number of calories.

Collagen

Collagen is a building block for cell structures and maintains firmness, such as that of your skin. Therefore, CAM practitioners speculate that collagen could also help improve the impermeability of the intestines. Bone broth is an extremely popular way to get collagen in the food you eat. It's easy to make and full of nutrition. Boil up and then simmer some bones, such as from a rotisserie chicken, with apple cider vinegar, for about 8 hours. Then drink as is or use in soups and stews.

Ginger

Ginger has been used in ancient medicine for thousands of years. It has warming and healing properties and has been associated with relief of arthritis and other inflammatory disorders. Use the fresh root or the dried and powdered form in a range of Indian and Chinese-style recipes.

L-Glutamine

L-glutamine is an important amino acid that the body uses in large amounts. It contributes to health in a number of ways, including:

- Improves gastrointestinal health because it is a vital nutrient that rebuilds and repairs

- Helps heal ulcers and leaky gut by boosting impermeability

- Serves as an essential neurotransmitter within the brain that helps with memory, focus and concentration, thus combatting 'memory fog', which often accompanies autoimmune disorders and arthritic conditions like fibromyalgia

- Improves IBS and diarrhea by balancing mucus production, which results in healthy bowel movements

- Promotes muscle growth and decreases muscle wastage, which happens as we age

- Helps maintain endurance during workouts

- Boosts metabolism

- Helps detoxify the body all the way down to the cellular level

- Improves athletic performance and recovery from endurance exercise

- Cuts cravings for sugar and for alcoholic beverages

- Improves blood sugar levels, important in relation to metabolic syndrome, pre-diabetes and diabetes

Natural sources include meat and poultry. Vegetable sources include:

- Beets

- Brussels sprouts

- Cabbage

- Carrots

- Kale

- Lentils, peas, beans and legumes

- Soybeans, tofu

- Spinach

Other main sources of L-glutamine include:

- Eggs, especially the whites

- Whole grains including oats, wheat germ and products made from whole wheat, quinoa, millet and brown rice.

- Nuts and nut butters, such as peanuts and peanut butter, almonds, pistachios, walnuts

- Seeds, such as pumpkin seeds and sunflower seeds

In most cases, people get more than enough L-glutamine via their ordinary diet. However, supplements are available and are recommended for people who have had surgery, especially gastrointestinal surgery. They are also given to people with extensive traumatic injuries and to cancer patients. High-endurance athletes will also use amino acid supplements that include L-glutamine.

If you are going to use a supplement, be sure to read the instructions and contraindications. Those with cirrhosis, liver disorders, epilepsy, and manic disorder should avoid it.

Licorice Root

Licorice root, which gives its flavor to black licorice, helps balance cortisol levels in the body and improves acid production in the stomach. It is also said to support the maintenance of the mucosal lining of the stomach. This herb is especially beneficial if someone's leaky gut is being caused by emotional stress. It is also used to treat diabetes.

However, it is important to note that licorice is a powerful herb which can have side effects even in small amounts. If you have heart health issues, high blood pressure, are on blood thinners, have kidney or liver issues, or are planning to have surgery, taking licorice can be risky.

Omega-3

As we discussed above, Omega-3 is anti-inflammatory and can soothe the gut. Oil also helps form an impermeable barrier, which can prevent leakage.

Omega-3 should not be taken if you have heart issues or are allergic to fish or shellfish. If you have the following health issues, you should avoid fish oil supplements:

- Bipolar disorder

- Depression

- Diabetes

- Heart issues

- High blood pressure

- HIV/AIDS

- Immune system disorders

- Liver disease

Quercetin

Quercetin is a plant pigment (flavonoid) which is found in many plants and foods, including:

- Apples

- Berries

- Buckwheat

- Green tea

- Gingko biloba

- St. John's Wort

- Onions

- Red wine

It is used for heart disease, diabetes, hay fever, peptic ulcer, inflammation, asthma, gout, viral infections, and chronic fatigue syndrome (CFS). Quercetin is also used to increase endurance and improve athletic performance. Large doses can cause kidney damage.

Turmeric

Turmeric is a bright yellow spice that has been used in Ayurvedic (traditional Indian) medicine for about 5,000 years. Turmeric is tasty, and adds an interesting flavor to Indian foods and rice dishes. It can be used in its fresh form, as a root, or dried and powdered.

Other supplements

Digestive enzymes and organic salts can also promote healthy digestion.

Digestive enzymes

There are eight primary digestive enzymes, each designed to help break down different types of food:

- Protease: Digests protein

- Amylase: Digests carbohydrates

- Lipase: Digests fats

- Cellulase: Breaks down fiber

- Maltase: Converts complex sugars from whole grains into glucose

- Lactase: Digests milk sugar (lactose) in dairy products

- Phytase: Helps with overall digestion, especially in extracting B vitamins

- Sucrase: Digesting most sugars

Your saliva is mainly made up of amylase. As the food passes through your system, protein is broken down by protease. Then the food passes to the small intestine, where the other enzymes do the rest.

In a normally functioning small intestine, the nutrients from your food are absorbed into your bloodstream through millions of tiny villi in the wall of your gut.

Think of them as the pile of a shag carpet.

However, in a leaky gut with low levels of enzymes, you will experience various symptoms, such as gas, bloating, acid reflux and more. Even if you do not have a leaky gut, your digestive enzyme production diminishes with age. This being the case, boosting your enzyme levels is a good idea and can also take the burden off your leaky gut.

Enzyme-rich foods include:

- Avocado

- Bee pollen

- Coconut oil

- Dairy products with live cultures

- Extra virgin olive oil

- Grapes

- Kiwi

- Mango

- Papaya

- Pineapple

If you've ever tried to make a Jell-O salad with kiwi or pineapple, you will know it doesn't work. This is because the high level of enzymes break down or basically start to digest the gelatin before it ever sets, so you can see how powerful these foods can be.

Other suggestions for boosting your enzymes are to:

- Eat a range of raw fruits and vegetables

- Don't overeat

- Chew slowly and thoroughly

- Avoid chewing gum, which stimulates enzyme

production because it thinks the body is getting food, but then they go to waste

Organic Salts

Organic salts, or tissue salts, are vital minerals that perform many functions in the body. They are commonly referred to as electrolytes and need to be replenished regularly for the body to perform all of its essential functions.

Organic salts include calcium, sodium, potassium, magnesium and phosphorous, on their own and in various combinations with one another. Phosphorous helps repair cells and tissues and could be very beneficial for leaky gut syndrome. A homeopath can help you with organic salts, but always try to get them through the food you eat first, rather than supplements.

If your stomach is very acidic, try:

- Apples

- Apricots

- Asparagus

- Carrots

- Grapes

- Peaches

- Raspberries

- Strawberries

If you often get cramps or heartburn, try:

- Bananas

- Figs

- Green leafy vegetables

- Lentils

- Oranges

- Walnuts

If you tend to have a nervous stomach, try eating more:

- Apples

- Broccoli

- Cauliflower

- Dates

- Garlic

- Guavas

- Lemons

- Oats

- Olives

- Onions

Hydrochloric Acid Supplements

The stomach produces hydrochloric acid to help digest food and also kill many potentially harmful bugs that could be in it. However, if acid levels aren't strong enough, it will be harder for the food to break down, leading to poor absorption of nutrients. It can also mean delayed emptying of the stomach, which can lead to a range of uncomfortable digestive symptoms.

If you think you might have a low level of hydrochloric acid, avoid drinking liquids with your meals. If that still doesn't work, try a supplement. Apple cider vinegar is commonly used to help lose weight but it can also aid digestion and relieve arthritis symptoms.

If you still don't seem to have enough stomach acid, there are a number of supplements available on the market that you can take with each meal. Finding the optimal dose can take some time and experimentation. You can take it one pill at a time until you get to the point where you start to feel like you have heartburn. In this case, take one less pill and track how you feel in your food diary.

Pure water

We should drink 8 eight-ounce glasses of fresh water every day. The trouble with this is that not all water is created equal.

Tap water has a variety of minerals in it depending on where you live. Some water is 'hard', with a great deal of minerality, while other water is termed soft.

In addition, tap is often treated with chlorine and fluoride, the former to prevent bacteria in the water, and the latter added to improve dental health. Both of these minerals have been suggested as possible causes of leaky gut, malabsorption of nutrients, and damage to the metabolism. Scientists who compared countries which did not fluoridate the water with those which did had far fewer obese people and ones suffering from digestive disorders.

Plus, if you have a leaky gut, drinking a lot of liquid will only increase the chance of leakage. Having said that, water is your best beverage of choice compared to soda, fruit juice, or other sugary drinks, and is definitely better for you than energy drinks and alcohol.

The trouble with bottled water is that some of it can be even less pure than what's already coming out of your tap, plus you have to lug it back and forth from the market. Invest in a filter like Pur that you put on your tap, or a couple of filtering jugs. Change the filters regularly according to the instructions. When used correctly, the filters can remove nearly 100% of the impurities in the water.

Save large 2-liter bottles and keep a supply of filtered water ready any time you need it. Buy a stainless steel water bottle for each member of the family so they can always have filtered water with them. Drink a little throughout the day to stay hydrated. Don't drink too much as one time, especially before or during a meal.

For people trying to lose weight who fill up on water to try to feel full so they will eat less, do it 2 hours after a meal so you don't interfere with your digestion.

Drinking before bedtime can be problematic because you may have to wake up several times in the middle of the night to urinate, so judge your consumption accordingly. If you have to urinate often at night, consider avoiding liquids after 9pm and try bladder training.

Water is an essential part of blood, filtration of the blood to remove toxins, and the digestive process, but impurities could be contribution to your leaky gut. Start drinking more water which you have filtered and note any changes in your symptoms in your food journal.

Conclusion

Leaky gut has only recently been started to be recognized by mainstream doctors, in the same that they ignored Lyme disease and fibromyalgia for decades until there was enough medical evidence to demonstrate that these symptoms were not all in people's minds, but were actually a sign of a genuine medical condition.

In the case of leaky gut, we can't be certain if it is a condition of its own, or associated with other medical conditions. But one thing is for sure. We don't want to sit around being ill and miserable until medical professionals finally start paying attention to us and taking our complaints seriously.

CAM practitioners such as homeopaths, naturopaths, Ayurvedic and traditional Chinese medicine practitioners work with people suffering from leaky gut and offer them safe, effective relief through food, drink, herbs and supplements, and lifestyle measures.

If you've been struggling with a range of digestive issues and unexplained symptoms, start a food journal. Then review what you've learned in this guide and start putting it into practice. Note down the foods you've added to your menus, and the ones you've removed and the changes experienced from each one – good and bad. Try an anti-inflammatory diet and healing foods. Then see what a difference they make to your health.

5-Point Action Plan: Recover From Your Leaky Gut

1-RECOGNIZE the symptoms
2-REMOVE foods and factors that damage the gut
3-REPLACE the damaging foods with healing foods
4-REPAIR your leaky gut with specific herbs and supplements
5-REBALANCE your gut flora with prebiotics and probiotics and helpful enzymes

1-RECOGNIZE YOUR SYMPTOMS AND DECIDE IF THEY COULD BE RELATED TO A LEAKY GUT:
-Digestive issues such as gas, bloating, diarrhea, constipation
-Depression
-Fatigue, generally feeling ill
-Muscle aches
-Inflammation such as redness, heat, pain, and swelling.

2-REMOVE FOODS KNOWN TO CAUSE LEAKY GUT
+Cow's milk and products made from it
+Whole grain wheat and glutens
+Tap water with chlorine and/or fluoride
+Sugar and salt
+Artificial sweeteners, colorings, preservatives
+Alcoholic beverages

3-REPLACE BAD FOODS WITH HEALING ONES
+Olive Oil
+Cherries, Berries
+Walnuts
+Bell peppers
+Ginger
+Turmeric
+Salmon and fatty fish/omega-3s
+Green leafy veggies and cruciferous veggies

4-REPAIR YOUR GUT WITH HERBS AND SUPPLEMENTS
+Aloe vera
+Butyrate
+Collagen
+Ginger
+L-glutamine
+Licorice Root
+Omega-3s
+Quercetin
+Turmeric

5-REBALANCE YOUR GUT FLORA
+Prebiotics
+Probiotics
+Digestive enzymes
+Organic Salts
+Hydrochloric acid supplements
+Reduce Stress

It takes time to find the right mix of foods to eat and those to avoid, but finding the balance could be the permanent fix to your unexplained sickness. Wouldn't that be great! To your best self!

Resources

Leaky Gut Syndrome

http://www.webmd.com/digestive-disorders/features/leaky-gut-syndrome

Leaky Gut Syndrome

http://www.nhs.uk/conditions/leaky-gut-syndrome/Pages/Introduction.aspx

Fish Oil Side Effects and Interactions

http://www.webmd.com/vitamins-supplements/ingredientmono-993-FISH+OIL.aspx?activeIngredientId=993&activeIngredientName=FISH+OIL&source=2

L-Glutamine

http://www.webmd.com/vitamins-supplements/ingredientmono-878-glutamine.aspx?activeingredientid=878&

Quercetin

http://www.webmd.com/vitamins-supplements/ingredientmono-294-QUERCETIN.aspx?activeIngredientId=294&activeIngredientName=QUERCETIN&source=2

Butyrate

http://bodyecology.com/articles/add-these-fiber-rich-foods-to-your-diet-to-fight-inflammation

Licorice Root

http://www.webmd.com/vitamins-supplements/ingredientmono-881-Licorice+root+LICORICE.aspx?activeIngredientId=881&activeIngredientName=Licorice+root+(LICORICE)&source=2

Other Health and Fitness Books by This Author

If you would like to read more about Senior Health and Fitness, here is a list of the titles, CreateSpace links and descriptions:

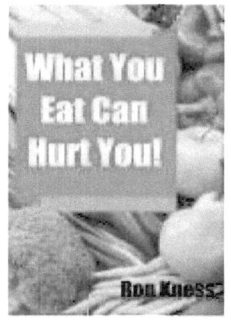

What You Eat Can Hurt You

https://www.createspace.com/4963196

Do you know that certain foods increase your risk for inflammation, disease and illness? It's true! And certain foods can help cure and heal you if you do get sick. Knowing which foods to eat and which ones to avoid empowers you to manage your own health.

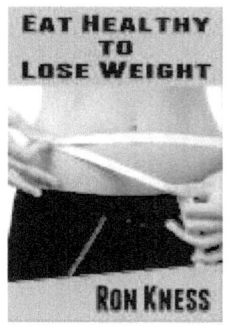

Eat Healthy to Lose Weight

https://www.createspace.com/4962939

As you read through our book, we show you which foods you should and should not be eating to reach your weight loss goal, along with discussing how to maintain your weight loss and stay within a few pounds of your goal weight. Banish the weight you keep gaining back each time by learning how to live a healthy lifestyle.

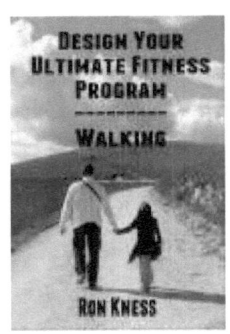 Design Your Ultimate Fitness Program - Walking

https://www.createspace.com/5252272

In my book Design Your Ultimate Fitness Program – Walking, we discuss the considerations that need to be made when designing a custom walking program, along with:

• Equipment needed
• Wearable technology you can use to track your walking
• And how to make walking more challenging

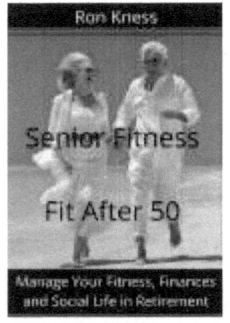 Senior Fitness – Fit After 50: Learn How to Manage Your Fitness, Finances and Social Life in Retirement

https://www.createspace.com/5474751

Inside you will discover answers to your most pressing questions:
• What do I need to know about downsizing my home?
• What are the best tips for staying healthy as you approach your 50's?
• When should I start planning for retirement?
• I am worried about being lonely once I retire, do others feel the same?
• Is it worthwhile to carry two homes during retirement?
And more…

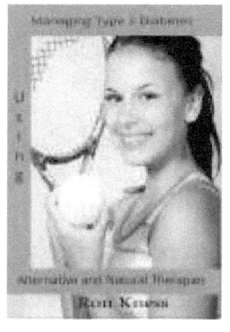

Managing Type 2 Diabetes Using Alternative And Natural Therapies

https://www.createspace.com/5401244

While Type 2 diabetes can be managed medically, there are many alternative natural and holistic methods of therapy and treatment that can further enhance quality of life and minimize the effects of this disease. In this book, I discuss 12 different types, including yoga, reflexology and acupuncture to name just three.

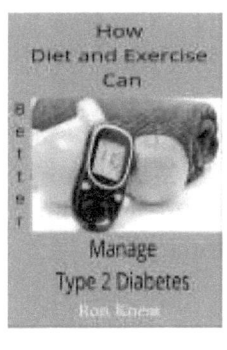

How Diet and Exercise Can Better Manage Type 2 Diabetes

https://www.createspace.com/5404845

Of the different types of diabetes, only Type 2 can be reversed. In my book How Diet and Exercise Can Better Manage Type 2 Diabetes, we reveal the three things you can do to best manage your disease, including:
• Diet
• Exercise
• Weight management

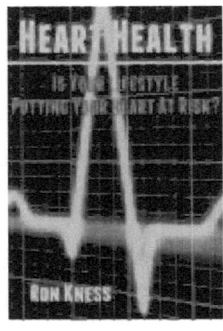

Heart Health: Is Your Lifestyle Putting Your Heart at Risk?

https://www.createspace.com/5464020

In my ebook Is Your Lifestyle Putting Your Heart At Risk? we discuss the six greatest risks to your heart and the lifestyle changes you can make to mitigate them.

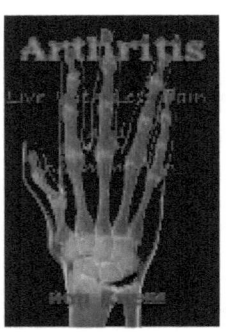

Arthritis – Live Wth Less Pain and Inflammation: Tips and Techniques You Can Use to Lessen the Pain and Inflammation

https://www.createspace.com/5457441

Discover Simple Tips & Information That Will Help Reduce The Painful Symptoms Of Arthritis!

You learn things like:
• Simple and effective information that will help you manage the pain and inflammation that comes along with arthritis, so that you can live an active, full life without debilitating pain.
• The different types of arthritis, their symptoms and how to alleviate their painful side effects.
• The pros and cons of over-the-counter arthritis medications, plus simple tips that will help you know how to choose the right supplements.
• Free, yet effective ways to get relief from arthritis pain and inflammation, so you don't have to suffer anymore.

the effects arthritis can have significant impact on your physical and mental well-being, but this books shows you how to overcome its painful symptoms and live life relatively pain free.

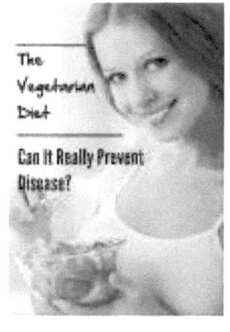

The Vegetarian Diet – Can It Really Prevent Disease?

https://www.createspace.com/5519874

Is a vegetarian diet right for you? Multiple studies have shown over and over that a vegetarian diet goes along way in preventing certain chronic diseases, such as:

• Heart Disease
• Cancer
• Diverticulitis
• Type 2 Diabetes
• Hypertension
• Obesity
• Kidney Failure

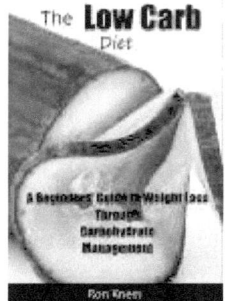

The Low Carb Diet: A Beginner's Guide to Weight Loss Through Carbohydrate Management

https://www.createspace.com/5416348

In my book "The Low-Carb Diet – A Beginners' Guide to Weight Loss Through Carbohydrate Management", I reveal a successful method of losing weight based in part on the amount and type of carbohydrates you consume.

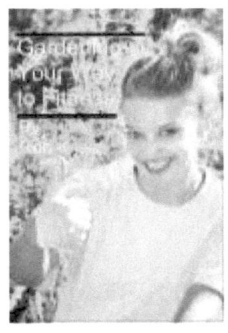

Gardening Your Way to Fitness: The Fun Way to Get Fit and Provide Beauty and Healthful Bounty for Your Family

https://www.createspace.com/5459564

The gym is a great place to stay fit during the colder seasons, but once the temperature turns warmer you want to spend more time outside. Plus, you'll have the benefit of fresh wholesome produce to enjoy by growing vegetables in your backyard garden.

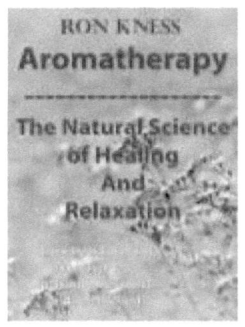

Aromatherapy - The Science of Healing and Relaxation: Learn How Essential Oils Elicit The Relaxation Response And Alter Mood

https://www.createspace.com/5714434

In my book Aromatherapy – The Science of Healing and Relaxation, we reveal the natural holistics methods you can use to heal the body from certain medical issues and to relive stress through relaxation. In particular we talk about:
• Aromatherapy - what it is and how it works
• Essential Oils – how the effects of certain aromas differs from others
• Recipes – how to make your own essential oil combinations

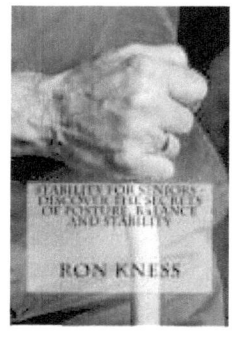

Stability for Seniors: Discover the Secrets of Posture, Balance and Stability

https://www.createspace.com/6096479

Many people sacrifice their health in pursuit of their career. They are so busy making a living that they neglect to make a life. The excuse that they do not have time to exercise is tossed about so frequently that they end up letting their health and fitness slide.

If you are not regularly active, you will have muscular atrophy over time. Your flexibility will decrease. Your core strength will diminish. As time progresses, you will be less limber and more rigid.

This is exactly how people age poorly. It's a process that has snowballed over time.

Only with regular exercise and a healthy diet can you have a body that is fit and has the ability to almost reverse aging.

If you have neglected your health for years and life seems to be a chore now because you can't get around without assistance, do not feel dejected.

You can remedy the situation. You can restore the strength, balance and stamina that you have lost. It is never too late to become what you might have been.

This guide will show you exactly what you need to do to restore your balance, strengthen your core and give you the ability to live life to its fullest. Read how …

About the Author

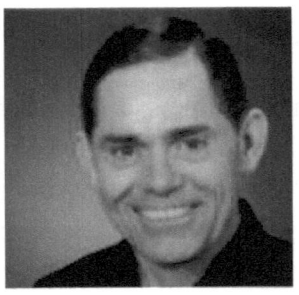

I grew up in Central Minnesota, where my parents owned and operated a fishing resort. Once out of high school I tried a couple of semesters of college, only to quit halfway through the Spring term; I decided at that time that college wasn't for me.

Then I decided to follow my father's previous occupation as an auto mechanic. I graduated from a two-year of vocational training course and worked as a mechanic for five years. While in vocational training, I decided to join the National Guard where I eventually ended up working full-time for 32 years.

So how does all of this relate to writing? In one of my leadership schools, the instructor, who was an English teacher at a juvenile detention center, presented writing to me in a whole new way - a way that started to develop my interest in working with words.

I eventually went back to college on the GI Bill while I was working and earned my Bachelor's degree in Business Administration. Taking a class or two per semester at night and on weekends took me seven years to complete my degree.

Fast forward about 40 years and I now have published over 75 books on Amazon for Kindle, CreateSpace and other publishing platforms.

Besides my own writing, I also ghostwrite ebooks, reports, articles, blogs and do Kindle conversions for clients on a variety of topics.

Today my wife and I are retired from our careers and live in Gold Canyon, AZ. I now write as a retirement business where you'll find me happily sitting in my office typing away on my laptop as I work on my next book or ghostwriting project . . . that is if we are not traveling on a cruise ship - our new-found mode of travel.